EASY PCOS DIET COOKBOOK

Nourishing Recipes and Meal Plans to Manage PCOS Effortlessly

Dr Lily Morgan

COPYRIGHT PAGE

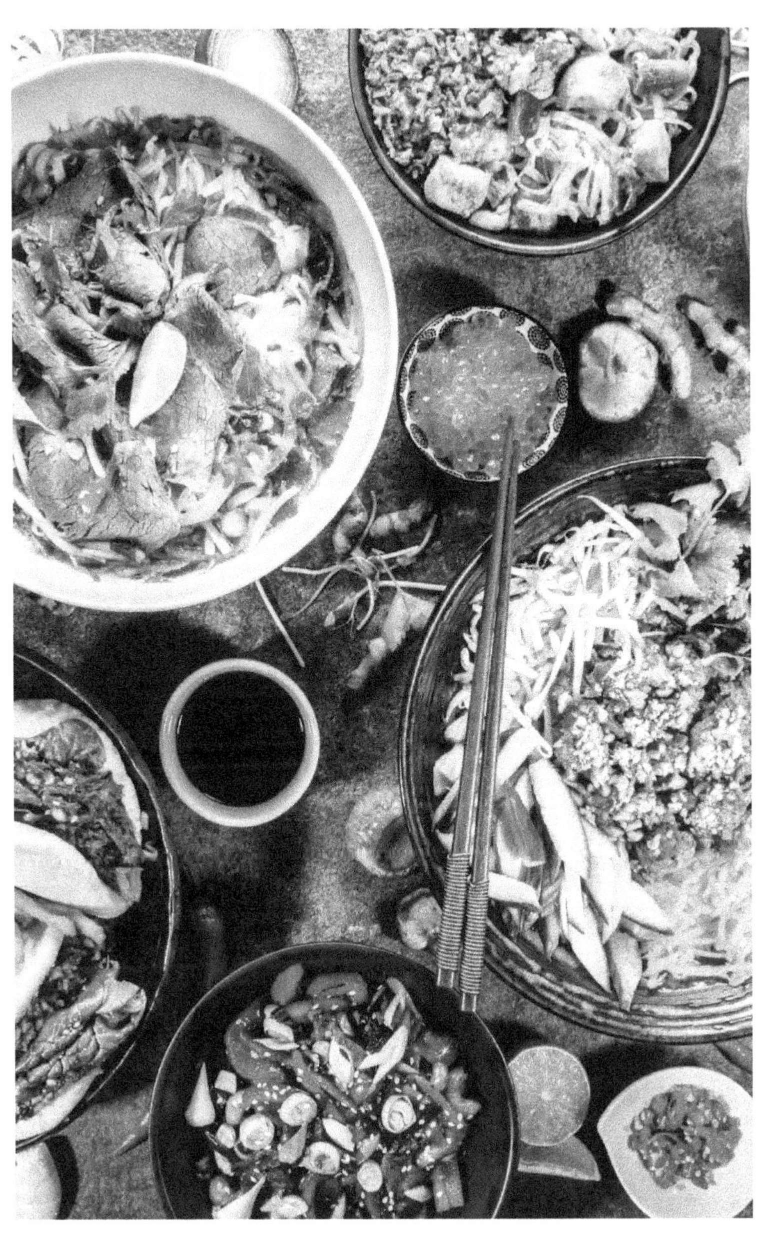

TABLE OF CONTENTS

Chapter 5: Snacks and Appetizers 70

INTRODUCTION

P COS is a multifaceted disorder characterized by hormonal imbalances and the development of small cysts on the ovaries. Its exact cause remains elusive, but research suggests a combination of genetic and environmental factors, insulin resistance, and elevated androgen levels play significant roles. By shedding light on the intricacies of PCOS, we empower individuals to take control of their health through dietary interventions.

The Impact of Diet on PCOS Symptoms

Diet plays a crucial role in managing PCOS symptoms and promoting hormonal balance. Certain food choices can exacerbate insulin resistance, inflammation, and hormonal imbalances, while others can alleviate these issues. By adopting an easy PCOS diet, individuals can make informed choices that support their well-being and minimize the impact of PCOS symptoms on their daily lives.

The Benefits of Following an Easy PCOS Diet

Embracing an easy PCOS diet can offer a myriad of benefits beyond symptom management. By focusing on whole, nutrient-dense foods, individuals can enhance their overall health, boost energy levels, regulate menstrual cycles, improve fertility, manage weight, reduce inflammation, and decrease the risk of long-term complications associated with PCOS. This chapter explores the extensive benefits that can be achieved through dietary modifications.

Navigating the PCOS Diet Journey

Embarking on a PCOS diet journey can be overwhelming, especially for those who are new to the concept. This section provides practical tips and guidance to ensure a smooth and successful transition. From meal planning and grocery shopping to navigating social situations and staying motivated, we offer strategies to help individuals overcome obstacles and stay on track with their dietary goals.

Equipping Your Kitchen for Success

A well-stocked kitchen is an essential component of any successful dietary journey. In this section, we provide a comprehensive list of pantry staples and kitchen equipment recommendations to support individuals in preparing PCOS-friendly meals. From high-quality oils and grains to essential tools and gadgets, we guide readers in creating a PCOS-friendly culinary haven that fosters creativity and enjoyment.

By immersing ourselves in the foundational knowledge provided in this introductory chapter, we establish a solid understanding of PCOS and its intricate relationship with diet. This knowledge serves as a strong foundation for the subsequent chapters, where we explore a wide array of delicious and easy-to-prepare recipes specifically designed to support individuals with PCOS. So, let's embark on this journey together, empowering ourselves with the tools and knowledge to embrace a healthy and fulfilling lifestyle despite the challenges of PCOS.

Chapter 1: 30-Day Meal Plan

This 30-day meal plan incorporates the provided recipes for each meal and offers a variety of options for breakfast, lunch, dinner, snacks, desserts, and smoothies. You can adjust the plan to suit your preferences and dietary needs

Week 1:

Day 1:

Breakfast: Fluffy Almond Flour Pancakes

Lunch: Grilled Chicken Salad with Lemon Dressing

Dinner: Baked Lemon Herb Chicken

Snack: Guacamole with Veggie Sticks

Dessert: Flourless Chocolate Cake

Smoothie: Green Detox Smoothie

Day 2:

Breakfast: Veggie Egg Muffins

Lunch: Quinoa and Roasted Vegetable Salad

Dinner: Shrimp Stir-Fry with Vegetables

Snack: Roasted Chickpeas

Dessert: Berry Chia Pudding

Smoothie: Turmeric Golden Milk

Day 3:

Breakfast: Chia Seed Pudding with Berries

Lunch: Turkey and Avocado Lettuce Wraps

Dinner: Spaghetti Squash with Meatballs

Snack: Greek Yogurt Dip with Fresh Veggies

Dessert: Almond Butter Cookies

Smoothie: Berry Blast Smoothie

Day 4:

Breakfast: Quinoa Breakfast Bowl

Lunch: Cauliflower Fried Rice

Dinner: Baked Salmon with Dill Sauce

Snack: Cucumber and Hummus Roll-Ups

Dessert: Greek Yogurt Berry Parfait

Smoothie: Iced Herbal Tea with Citrus

Day 5:

Breakfast: Avocado and Egg Toast

Lunch: Lentil Soup with Spinach

Dinner: Turkey Chili with Sweet Potatoes

Snack: Baked Sweet Potato Fries

Dessert: Pumpkin Spice Muffins

Smoothie: Cucumber and Mint Infused Water

Day 6:

Breakfast: Greek Yogurt Parfait with Granola

Lunch: Tuna and White Bean Salad

Dinner: Roasted Cauliflower Steaks

Snack: Caprese Skewers

Dessert: Coconut Macaroons

Smoothie: Energizing Matcha Latte

Day 7:

Breakfast: Spinach and Mushroom Omelette

Lunch: Zucchini Noodles with Pesto

Dinner: Mexican Stuffed Zucchini Boats

Snack: Energy Bites with Nuts and Dates

Dessert: Baked Apples with Cinnamon

Smoothie: Refreshing Watermelon Cooler

Week 2:

Day 8:

Breakfast: Coconut Flour Banana Bread

Lunch: Mediterranean Chickpea Salad

Dinner: Lemon Garlic Shrimp and Broccoli

Snack: Kale Chips

Dessert: Chocolate Avocado Mousse

Smoothie: Blueberry Lemonade

Day 9:

Breakfast: Sweet Potato Hash with Poached Eggs

Lunch: Salmon and Quinoa Bowl

Dinner: Quinoa-Stuffed Bell Peppers

Snack: Spinach and Artichoke Dip

Dessert: Lemon Poppy Seed Loaf

Smoothie: Spiced Apple Cider

Day 10:

Breakfast: Green Smoothie Bowl

Lunch: Greek-Style Stuffed Bell Peppers

Dinner: Baked Cod with Tomato and Olive Relish

Snack: Zucchini Fritters with Tzatziki Sauce

Dessert: Vanilla Berry Nice Cream

Smoothie: Coconut Water Electrolyte Drink

Day 11:

Breakfast: Fluffy Almond Flour Pancakes

Lunch: Grilled Chicken Salad with Lemon Dressing

Dinner: Baked Lemon Herb Chicken

Snack: Guacamole with Veggie Sticks

Dessert: Flourless Chocolate Cake

Smoothie: Green Detox Smoothie

Day 12:

Breakfast: Veggie Egg Muffins

Lunch: Quinoa and Roasted Vegetable Salad

Dinner: Shrimp Stir-Fry with Vegetables

Snack: Roasted Chickpeas

Dessert: Berry Chia Pudding

Smoothie: Turmeric Golden Milk

Day 13:

Breakfast: Chia Seed Pudding with Berries

Lunch: Turkey and Avocado Lettuce Wraps

Dinner: Spaghetti Squash with Meatballs

Snack: Greek Yogurt Dip with Fresh Veggies

Dessert: Almond Butter Cookies

Smoothie: Berry Blast Smoothie

Day 14:

Breakfast: Quinoa Breakfast Bowl

Lunch: Cauliflower Fried Rice

Dinner: Baked Salmon with Dill Sauce

Snack: Cucumber and Hummus Roll-Ups

Dessert: Greek Yogurt Berry Parfait

Smoothie: Iced Herbal Tea with Citrus

Week 3:

Day 15:

Breakfast: Avocado and Egg Toast

Lunch: Lentil Soup with Spinach

Dinner: Turkey Chili with Sweet Potatoes

Snack: Baked Sweet Potato Fries

Dessert: Pumpkin Spice Muffins

Smoothie: Cucumber and Mint Infused Water

Day 16:

Breakfast: Greek Yogurt Parfait with Granola

Lunch: Tuna and White Bean Salad

Dinner: Roasted Cauliflower Steaks

Snack: Caprese Skewers

Dessert: Coconut Macaroons

Smoothie: Energizing Matcha Latte

Day 17:

Breakfast: Spinach and Mushroom Omelette

Lunch: Zucchini Noodles with Pesto

Dinner: Mexican Stuffed Zucchini Boats

Snack: Energy Bites with Nuts and Dates

Dessert: Baked Apples with Cinnamon

Smoothie: Refreshing Watermelon Cooler

Day 18:

Breakfast: Coconut Flour Banana Bread

Lunch: Mediterranean Chickpea Salad

Dinner: Lemon Garlic Shrimp and Broccoli

Snack: Kale Chips

Dessert: Chocolate Avocado Mousse

Smoothie: Blueberry Lemonade

Day 19:

Breakfast: Sweet Potato Hash with Poached Eggs

Lunch: Salmon and Quinoa Bowl

Dinner: Quinoa-Stuffed Bell Peppers

Snack: Spinach and Artichoke Dip

Dessert: Lemon Poppy Seed Loaf

Smoothie: Spiced Apple Cider

Day 20:

Breakfast: Green Smoothie Bowl

Lunch: Greek-Style Stuffed Bell Peppers

Dinner: Baked Cod with Tomato and Olive Relish

Snack: Zucchini Fritters with Tzatziki Sauce

Dessert: Vanilla Berry Nice Cream

Smoothie: Coconut Water Electrolyte Drink

Day 21:

Breakfast: Fluffy Almond Flour Pancakes

Lunch: Grilled Chicken Salad with Lemon Dressing

Dinner: Baked Lemon Herb Chicken

Snack: Guacamole with Veggie Sticks

Dessert: Flourless Chocolate Cake

Smoothie: Green Detox Smoothie

Week 4:

Day 22:

Breakfast: Veggie Egg Muffins

Lunch: Quinoa and Roasted Vegetable Salad

Dinner: Shrimp Stir-Fry with Vegetables

Snack: Roasted Chickpeas

Dessert: Berry Chia Pudding

Smoothie: Turmeric Golden Milk

Day 23:

Breakfast: Chia Seed Pudding with Berries

Lunch: Turkey and Avocado Lettuce Wraps

Dinner: Spaghetti Squash with Meatballs

Snack: Greek Yogurt Dip with Fresh Veggies

Dessert: Almond Butter Cookies

Smoothie: Berry Blast Smoothie

Day 24:

Breakfast: Quinoa Breakfast Bowl

Lunch: Cauliflower Fried Rice

Dinner: Baked Salmon with Dill Sauce

Snack: Cucumber and Hummus Roll-Ups

Dessert: Greek Yogurt Berry Parfait

Smoothie: Iced Herbal Tea with Citrus

Day 25:

Breakfast: Avocado and Egg Toast

Lunch: Lentil Soup with Spinach

Dinner: Turkey Chili with Sweet Potatoes

Snack: Baked Sweet Potato Fries

Dessert: Pumpkin Spice Muffins

Smoothie: Cucumber and Mint Infused Water

Day 26:

Breakfast: Greek Yogurt Parfait with Granola

Lunch: Tuna and White Bean Salad

Dinner: Roasted Cauliflower Steaks

Snack: Caprese Skewers

Dessert: Coconut Macaroons

Smoothie: Energizing Matcha Latte

Day 27:

Breakfast: Spinach and Mushroom Omelette

Lunch: Zucchini Noodles with Pesto

Dinner: Mexican Stuffed Zucchini Boats

Snack: Energy Bites with Nuts and Dates

Dessert: Baked Apples with Cinnamon

Smoothie: Refreshing Watermelon Cooler

Day 28:

Breakfast: Coconut Flour Banana Bread

Lunch: Mediterranean Chickpea Salad

Dinner: Lemon Garlic Shrimp and Broccoli

Snack: Kale Chips

Dessert: Chocolate Avocado Mousse

Smoothie: Blueberry Lemonade

Day 29:

Breakfast: Sweet Potato Hash with Poached Eggs

Lunch: Salmon and Quinoa Bowl

Dinner: Quinoa-Stuffed Bell Peppers

Snack: Spinach and Artichoke Dip

Dessert: Lemon Poppy Seed Loaf

Smoothie: Spiced Apple Cider

Day 30:

Breakfast: Green Smoothie Bowl

Lunch: Greek-Style Stuffed Bell Peppers

Dinner: Baked Cod with Tomato and Olive Relish

Snack: Zucchini Fritters with Tzatziki Sauce

Dessert: Vanilla Berry Nice Cream

Smoothie: Coconut Water Electrolyte Drink

Chapter 2: Breakfast Recipes

In this chapter, you'll discover a variety of delicious and nutritious Breakfast Recipes to kickstart your day on a healthy note. These recipes are specifically designed to support a PCOS diet while providing you with a satisfying and energizing meal.

Fluffy Almond Flour Pancakes

Ingredients:

- 1 cup almond flour
- 2 tablespoons coconut flour
- 1 teaspoon baking powder
- 1/4 teaspoon salt
- 2 large eggs
- 1/4 cup almond milk
- 2 tablespoons honey or maple syrup
- 1 teaspoon vanilla extract
- Coconut oil or butter for cooking

Instructions:

1. In a mixing bowl, whisk together the almond flour, coconut flour, baking powder, and salt.
2. In a separate bowl, beat the eggs and then add almond milk, honey (or maple syrup), and vanilla extract. Mix well.
3. Combine the wet ingredients with the dry ingredients and stir until a smooth batter forms.
4. Heat a non-stick skillet or griddle over medium heat and lightly grease with coconut oil or butter.
5. Pour about 1/4 cup of batter onto the skillet for each pancake. Cook for 2-3 minutes until bubbles form on the surface, then flip and cook for another 1-2 minutes.
6. Repeat with the remaining batter, adding more oil or butter as needed.
7. Serve the fluffy almond flour pancakes warm with your favorite toppings like fresh berries, Greek yogurt, or a drizzle of honey.

Veggie Egg Muffins

Ingredients:

- 6 large eggs
- 1/4 cup milk (dairy or plant-based)
- 1/2 cup chopped bell peppers
- 1/2 cup chopped spinach
- 1/4 cup diced onions
- 1/4 cup grated cheddar cheese (optional)
- Salt and pepper to taste
- Cooking spray

Instructions:

1. Preheat your oven to 350°F (175°C) and lightly grease a muffin tin with cooking spray.
2. In a bowl, whisk together the eggs and milk until well combined. Season with salt and pepper.
3. Stir in the chopped bell peppers, spinach, onions, and grated cheddar cheese (if using).
4. Pour the egg mixture evenly into the prepared muffin tin, filling each cup about 3/4 full.
5. Bake for 18-20 minutes or until the egg muffins are set and slightly golden on top.

6. Remove from the oven and let them cool for a few minutes before removing them from the muffin tin.

7. Serve these veggie egg muffins as a convenient and protein-packed breakfast option. They can be enjoyed hot or cold and can be stored in the refrigerator for a few days.

Chia Seed Pudding with Berries

Ingredients:

- 1/4 cup chia seeds
- 1 cup unsweetened almond milk (or any milk of your choice)
- 1 tablespoon honey or maple syrup
- 1/2 teaspoon vanilla extract
- Fresh berries for topping

Instructions:

1. In a jar or bowl, combine the chia seeds, almond milk, honey (or maple syrup), and vanilla extract.

2. Stir well to make sure the chia seeds are fully immersed in the liquid.

3. Let the mixture sit for about 5 minutes, then stir
    again to prevent clumping.
4. Cover the jar or bowl and refrigerate for at least 2
    hours or overnight.
5. After the chia seeds have absorbed the liquid and
    the mixture has thickened to a pudding-like
    consistency, give it a final stir.
6. Serve the chia seed pudding in individual bowls or
    glasses and top with fresh berries.
7. Enjoy this nutritious and satisfying chia seed
    pudding as a delicious breakfast or snack option.

Quinoa Breakfast Bowl

Ingredients:

- 1 cup cooked quinoa
- 1/2 cup almond milk (or any milk of your choice)
- 1 tablespoon honey or maple syrup
- 1/2 teaspoon cinnamon
- 1/4 cup chopped nuts (e.g., almonds, walnuts)
- 1/4 cup fresh berries
- 1 tablespoon unsweetened coconut flakes (optional)

Instructions:

1. In a saucepan, warm the cooked quinoa with almond milk over medium heat.

2. Stir in the honey (or maple syrup) and cinnamon. Cook for 2-3 minutes until heated through.

3. Transfer the quinoa mixture to a bowl.

4. Top with chopped nuts, fresh berries, and unsweetened coconut flakes (if desired).

5. Feel free to customize your quinoa breakfast bowl with additional toppings such as sliced bananas, diced apples, or a dollop of Greek yogurt.

6. Enjoy this wholesome and protein-rich breakfast bowl to start your day on a nutritious note.

Avocado and Egg Toast

Ingredients:

- 2 slices of whole-grain bread, toasted
- 1 ripe avocado
- 2 large eggs
- Salt and pepper to taste
- Optional toppings: sliced tomatoes, microgreens, hot sauce

Instructions:

1. Slice the ripe avocado in half and remove the pit. Scoop out the flesh into a small bowl.
2. Mash the avocado with a fork until creamy, then season with salt and pepper to taste.
3. Spread the mashed avocado evenly onto the toasted bread slices.
4. In a non-stick skillet, fry the eggs to your desired doneness (e.g., sunny-side up, over-easy).
5. Carefully place one fried egg on each avocado toast.
6. Sprinkle with additional salt and pepper if desired and add optional toppings like sliced tomatoes, microgreens, or a drizzle of hot sauce.
7. Serve the avocado and egg toast as a satisfying and nourishing breakfast option.

Greek Yogurt Parfait with Granola

Ingredients:

- 1 cup plain Greek yogurt
- 1/4 cup granola (choose a variety without added sugars)
- 1/2 cup fresh berries

- 1 tablespoon honey or maple syrup (optional)

Instructions:

1. In a glass or bowl, layer half of the Greek yogurt.
2. Sprinkle half of the granola over the yogurt.
3. Add half of the fresh berries on top.
4. Repeat the layers with the remaining Greek yogurt, granola, and berries.
5. Drizzle with honey or maple syrup if desired for extra sweetness.
6. Enjoy this delightful and protein-packed Greek yogurt parfait as a healthy breakfast or snack.

Spinach and Mushroom Omelette

Ingredients:

- 3 large eggs
- 1 tablespoon milk (dairy or plant-based)
- 1/2 cup chopped spinach
- 1/4 cup sliced mushrooms
- 1/4 cup diced onions
- Salt and pepper to taste
- Cooking oil or butter

Instructions:

1. In a bowl, whisk together the eggs and milk. Season with salt and pepper.
2. Heat a non-stick skillet over medium heat and add a small amount of cooking oil or butter.
3. Sauté the chopped spinach, sliced mushrooms, and diced onions until they soften.
4. Pour the egg mixture over the cooked vegetables in the skillet.
5. Gently swirl the skillet to distribute the eggs and vegetables evenly.
6. Cook for a few minutes until the omelette is set around the edges.
7. Carefully flip or fold the omelette in half and continue cooking for another minute until the eggs are fully cooked.
8. Slide the spinach and mushroom omelette onto a plate and serve hot.
9. Pair this nutritious omelette with whole-grain toast or a side salad for a well-rounded breakfast.

Coconut Flour Banana Bread

Ingredients:

- 1/2 cup coconut flour
- 1/2 teaspoon baking soda
- 1/4 teaspoon salt
- 3 ripe bananas, mashed
- 4 large eggs
- 1/4 cup coconut oil, melted
- 1/4 cup honey or maple syrup
- 1 teaspoon vanilla extract
- Optional add-ins: chopped nuts, chocolate chips, dried fruits

Instructions:

1. Preheat your oven to 350°F (175°C) and grease a loaf pan.
2. In a bowl, whisk together the coconut flour, baking soda, and salt.
3. In a separate bowl, combine the mashed bananas, eggs, melted coconut oil, honey (or maple syrup), and vanilla extract. Mix well.

4. Add the wet ingredients to the dry ingredients and stir until a smooth batter forms.

5. If desired, fold in chopped nuts, chocolate chips, or dried fruits for added flavor and texture.

6. Pour the batter into the greased loaf pan and spread it evenly.

7. Bake for 45-50 minutes or until a toothpick inserted into the center comes out clean.

8. Remove the coconut flour banana bread from the oven and let it cool in the pan for a few minutes before transferring it to a wire rack to cool completely.

9. Slice and enjoy this moist and flavorful banana bread as a nutritious breakfast treat or snack.

Sweet Potato Hash with Poached Eggs

Ingredients:

- 1 large sweet potato, peeled and diced
- 1/2 red bell pepper, diced
- 1/2 green bell pepper, diced
- 1/4 cup diced onions

- 2 tablespoons olive oil
- 1/2 teaspoon paprika
- 1/2 teaspoon garlic powder
- Salt and pepper to taste
- 4 large eggs, poached

Instructions:

1. Heat olive oil in a skillet over medium heat.
2. Add the diced sweet potato, bell peppers, and onions to the skillet.
3. Sprinkle paprika, garlic powder, salt, and pepper over the vegetables.
4. Sauté for 10-12 minutes or until the sweet potatoes are tender and lightly browned.
5. While the sweet potato hash is cooking, prepare the poached eggs according to your preferred method.
6. Serve the sweet potato hash topped with poached eggs.
7. Season with additional salt and pepper if desired.
8. Enjoy this hearty and nutritious sweet potato hash with poached eggs for a satisfying breakfast or brunch.

Green Smoothie Bowl

Ingredients:

- 1 ripe banana
- 1 cup spinach leaves
- 1/2 cup frozen mango chunks
- 1/2 cup frozen pineapple chunks
- 1/2 cup almond milk (or any milk of your choice)
- Toppings: sliced fresh fruit, granola, chia seeds, shredded coconut

Instructions:

1. In a blender, combine the ripe banana, spinach leaves, frozen mango chunks, frozen pineapple chunks, and almond milk.
2. Blend until smooth and creamy, adding more almond milk if needed to reach the desired consistency.
3. Pour the green smoothie into a bowl.
4. Top with sliced fresh fruit, granola, chia seeds, and shredded coconut for added texture and flavor.

5. Enjoy this vibrant and nutrient-packed green smoothie bowl as a refreshing breakfast or snack option.

Chapter 3: Lunch Recipes

In this chapter, you'll discover a variety of delicious and nutritious Lunch Recipes to kickstart your day on a healthy note. These recipes are specifically designed to support a PCOS diet while providing you with a satisfying and energizing meal.

Grilled Chicken Salad with Lemon Dressing

Ingredients:

- 1 boneless, skinless chicken breast
- 2 cups mixed salad greens
- 1/4 cup cherry tomatoes, halved
- 1/4 cup cucumber, sliced
- 1/4 cup red onion, thinly sliced
- 2 tablespoons feta cheese, crumbled
- 1 tablespoon fresh parsley, chopped

For the Lemon Dressing:

- 2 tablespoons fresh lemon juice

- 1 tablespoon extra-virgin olive oil

- 1 teaspoon Dijon mustard

- Salt and pepper to taste

Instructions:

1. Preheat a grill or grill pan over medium heat.

2. Season the chicken breast with salt and pepper.

3. Grill the chicken for about 6-8 minutes per side or until cooked through. Allow it to rest for a few minutes before slicing.

4. In a large bowl, combine the salad greens, cherry tomatoes, cucumber, red onion, feta cheese, and parsley.

5. In a separate small bowl, whisk together the lemon juice, olive oil, Dijon mustard, salt, and pepper to make the dressing.

6. Drizzle the lemon dressing over the salad and toss to coat.

7. Slice the grilled chicken and place it on top of the salad.

8. Serve immediately and enjoy!

Quinoa and Roasted Vegetable Salad

Ingredients:

- 1 cup cooked quinoa
- 1 cup roasted vegetables (such as bell peppers, zucchini, and eggplant), diced
- 1/4 cup crumbled feta cheese
- 2 tablespoons chopped fresh basil
- 2 tablespoons extra-virgin olive oil
- 1 tablespoon balsamic vinegar
- Salt and pepper to taste

Instructions:

1. In a large bowl, combine the cooked quinoa, roasted vegetables, feta cheese, and basil.
2. In a small bowl, whisk together the olive oil, balsamic vinegar, salt, and pepper.
3. Drizzle the dressing over the quinoa and roasted vegetable mixture. Toss gently to combine.
4. Adjust the seasoning if needed.
5. Allow the salad to sit for a few minutes to let the flavors meld together.

6. Serve at room temperature or chilled. Enjoy this hearty and nutritious salad for breakfast!

Turkey and Avocado Lettuce Wraps

Ingredients:

- 4 large lettuce leaves (such as iceberg or butter lettuce)
- 8 ounces cooked turkey breast, sliced
- 1 avocado, pitted and sliced
- 1/2 cup cherry tomatoes, halved
- 1/4 cup red onion, thinly sliced
- 2 tablespoons fresh cilantro, chopped
- Juice of 1 lime
- Salt and pepper to taste

Instructions:

1. Place the lettuce leaves on a clean surface.
2. Layer the turkey slices, avocado slices, cherry tomatoes, red onion, and fresh cilantro on each lettuce leaf.
3. Squeeze lime juice over the fillings.
4. Sprinkle with salt and pepper to taste.

5. Roll up the lettuce leaves tightly, securing them with toothpicks if needed.

6. Slice each lettuce wrap in half diagonally.

7. Serve immediately and savor the combination of flavors and textures in this refreshing breakfast option.

Cauliflower Fried Rice

Ingredients:

- 1 medium head cauliflower, grated or processed into rice-like pieces
- 2 tablespoons coconut oil
- 2 cloves garlic, minced
- 1/2 cup frozen peas and carrots, thawed
- 2 green onions, chopped
- 2 large eggs, beaten
- 2 tablespoons low-sodium soy sauce or tamari
- 1 tablespoon sesame oil
- Salt and pepper to taste

Instructions:

1. Heat coconut oil in a large skillet or wok over medium heat.

2. Add the minced garlic and sauté for 1-2 minutes until fragrant.

3. Add the cauliflower rice, frozen peas and carrots, and chopped green onions to the skillet. Stir-fry for about 5 minutes until the vegetables are tender.

4. Push the cauliflower mixture to one side of the skillet and pour the beaten eggs into the empty side. Scramble the eggs until fully cooked.

5. Mix the scrambled eggs with the cauliflower mixture.

6. Stir in the soy sauce or tamari, sesame oil, salt, and pepper. Cook for an additional 1-2 minutes, ensuring everything is well combined and heated through.

7. Remove from heat and serve hot. This low-carb cauliflower fried rice is a satisfying and nutritious breakfast option.

Lentil Soup with Spinach

Ingredients:

- 1 cup dried green lentils, rinsed
- 4 cups vegetable broth
- 1 tablespoon olive oil
- 1 medium onion, chopped
- 2 cloves garlic, minced
- 2 carrots, diced
- 2 celery stalks, diced
- 1 teaspoon ground cumin
- 1 teaspoon ground coriander
- 1/2 teaspoon turmeric
- 4 cups fresh spinach leaves
- Salt and pepper to taste

Instructions:

1. In a large pot, bring the vegetable broth to a boil. Add the lentils and reduce the heat to a simmer. Cook for about 20-25 minutes or until the lentils are tender.

2. In a separate skillet, heat the olive oil over medium heat. Add the chopped onion, minced garlic, carrots,

and celery. Sauté until the vegetables are tender, about 5-7 minutes.

3. Stir in the ground cumin, ground coriander, and turmeric. Cook for an additional minute to toast the spices and enhance their flavors.

4. Transfer the sautéed vegetables to the pot with the lentils.

5. Add the fresh spinach leaves to the pot and stir until wilted.

6. Season with salt and pepper to taste.

7. Simmer the soup for an additional 5 minutes to allow the flavors to meld together.

8. Remove from heat and serve hot. This protein-packed lentil soup with spinach makes for a nourishing and hearty breakfast.

Tuna and White Bean Salad

Ingredients:

- 1 can (5 ounces) tuna in water, drained
- 1 can (15 ounces) white beans, rinsed and drained
- 1/4 cup red onion, finely chopped
- 1/4 cup fresh parsley, chopped

- 2 tablespoons lemon juice
- 2 tablespoons extra-virgin olive oil
- Salt and pepper to taste

Instructions:

1. In a large bowl, combine the drained tuna, white beans, red onion, and fresh parsley.
2. In a small bowl, whisk together the lemon juice, olive oil, salt, and pepper.
3. Pour the dressing over the tuna and white bean mixture. Gently toss to coat.
4. Adjust the seasoning if needed.
5. Allow the salad to chill in the refrigerator for at least 30 minutes to let the flavors marry together.
6. Serve chilled and enjoy this protein-rich breakfast salad.

Zucchini Noodles with Pesto

Ingredients:

- 2 medium zucchini, spiralized into noodles
- 1/4 cup homemade or store-bought pesto
- 1/4 cup cherry tomatoes, halved

- 2 tablespoons pine nuts, toasted

- Fresh basil leaves for garnish

- Salt and pepper to taste

Instructions:

1. Heat a skillet over medium heat and add the spiralized zucchini noodles. Sauté for about 2-3 minutes until the noodles are slightly softened.

2. Remove the skillet from heat and transfer the zucchini noodles to a large bowl.

3. Add the pesto to the bowl and toss to coat the noodles evenly.

4. Gently fold in the cherry tomatoes and toasted pine nuts.

5. Season with salt and pepper to taste.

6. Garnish with fresh basil leaves.

7. Serve immediately and relish in the fresh and vibrant flavors of this zucchini noodle dish.

Mediterranean Chickpea Salad

Ingredients:

- 1 can (15 ounces) chickpeas, rinsed and drained

- 1 cup cucumber, diced

- 1 cup cherry tomatoes, halved

- 1/4 cup red onion, thinly sliced

- 1/4 cup Kalamata olives, pitted and halved

- 2 tablespoons fresh parsley, chopped

- 2 tablespoons extra-virgin olive oil

- 1 tablespoon lemon juice

- 1 teaspoon dried oregano

- Salt and pepper to taste

Instructions:

1. In a large bowl, combine the chickpeas, cucumber, cherry tomatoes, red onion, Kalamata olives, and fresh parsley.

2. In a small bowl, whisk together the olive oil, lemon juice, dried oregano, salt, and pepper.

3. Drizzle the dressing over the chickpea salad. Toss gently to combine.

4. Adjust the seasoning if needed.

5. Allow the flavors to meld together by refrigerating the salad for at least 30 minutes.

6. Serve chilled and enjoy the Mediterranean-inspired
    flavors of this refreshing salad.

Salmon and Quinoa Bowl

Ingredients:

- 1 cup cooked quinoa
- 4 ounces cooked salmon fillet, flaked
- 1/2 cup steamed broccoli florets
- 1/4 cup shredded carrots
- 1/4 cup sliced cucumber
- 2 tablespoons soy sauce or tamari
- 1 tablespoon rice vinegar
- 1 teaspoon honey or maple syrup
- Sesame seeds for garnish

Instructions:

1. In a bowl, layer the cooked quinoa, flaked salmon,
    steamed broccoli florets, shredded carrots, and
    sliced cucumber.
2. In a small bowl, whisk together the soy sauce or
    tamari, rice vinegar, and honey or maple syrup to
    make the dressing.

3. Drizzle the dressing over the quinoa bowl.

4. Sprinkle with sesame seeds for garnish.

5. Serve at room temperature or chilled. This salmon and quinoa bowl is a nutrient-dense and satisfying breakfast option.

Greek-Style Stuffed Bell Peppers

Ingredients:

- 2 large bell peppers (any color), halved and seeded
- 1 cup cooked quinoa
- 1/2 cup cherry tomatoes, halved
- 1/4 cup Kalamata olives, pitted and chopped
- 1/4 cup crumbled feta cheese
- 2 tablespoons chopped fresh parsley
- 1 tablespoon lemon juice
- 1 tablespoon extra-virgin olive oil
- Salt and pepper to taste

Instructions:

1. Preheat the oven to 375°F (190°C).

2. Place the bell pepper halves on a baking sheet, cut side up.

3. In a bowl, combine the cooked quinoa, cherry tomatoes, Kalamata olives, feta cheese, chopped parsley, lemon juice, olive oil, salt, and pepper.

4. Spoon the quinoa mixture into each bell pepper half, filling them generously.

5. Bake in the preheated oven for about 20-25 minutes or until the bell peppers are tender and slightly charred.

6. Remove from the oven and let them cool for a few minutes before serving.

7. Enjoy these Greek-inspired stuffed bell peppers as a flavorful and wholesome breakfast.

Chapter 4: Dinner Recipes

In this chapter, we will explore a variety of delicious dinner recipes that are both nutritious and suitable for individuals with PCOS. These recipes are designed to help you maintain a balanced diet while enjoying flavorful meals. Let's dive into the wonderful world of dinner recipes!

Baked Lemon Herb Chicken

Ingredients:

- 4 boneless, skinless chicken breasts
- 2 tablespoons olive oil
- 1 lemon, juiced and zested
- 2 cloves garlic, minced
- 1 teaspoon dried thyme
- 1 teaspoon dried rosemary
- Salt and pepper to taste

Instructions:

1. Preheat the oven to 400°F (200°C) and line a baking dish with parchment paper.

2. In a small bowl, whisk together the olive oil, lemon juice, lemon zest, minced garlic, dried thyme, dried rosemary, salt, and pepper.

3. Place the chicken breasts in the prepared baking dish and pour the lemon herb mixture over them, ensuring they are evenly coated.

4. Bake the chicken for about 25-30 minutes or until cooked through and the internal temperature reaches 165°F (75°C).

5. Remove the chicken from the oven and let it rest for a few minutes before serving. Serve with a side of steamed vegetables or a salad.

Shrimp Stir-Fry with Vegetables

Ingredients:

- 1 pound shrimp, peeled and deveined
- 2 tablespoons olive oil
- 2 cloves garlic, minced
- 1 red bell pepper, sliced
- 1 yellow bell pepper, sliced
- 1 zucchini, sliced
- 1 cup broccoli florets

- 1 cup snap peas

- 2 tablespoons low-sodium soy sauce

- 1 tablespoon honey or maple syrup

- 1 teaspoon sesame oil

- Sesame seeds for garnish (optional)

Instructions:

1. Heat olive oil in a large skillet or wok over medium-high heat.

2. Add the minced garlic and sauté for about 1 minute until fragrant.

3. Add the shrimp to the skillet and cook for 2-3 minutes until they start to turn pink. Remove the shrimp from the skillet and set aside.

4. In the same skillet, add the sliced bell peppers, zucchini, broccoli florets, and snap peas. Stir-fry for about 5-6 minutes until the vegetables are tender-crisp.

5. In a small bowl, whisk together the soy sauce, honey or maple syrup, and sesame oil.

6. Return the cooked shrimp to the skillet and pour the sauce over the shrimp and vegetables. Stir-fry for an

additional 1-2 minutes until everything is well coated.

7. Remove from heat and sprinkle with sesame seeds if desired. Serve hot with steamed rice or cauliflower rice.

Spaghetti Squash with Meatballs

Ingredients:

- 1 spaghetti squash
- 1 pound lean ground beef or turkey
- 1/2 cup almond flour or breadcrumbs
- 1/4 cup grated Parmesan cheese
- 1 egg
- 1/4 cup chopped fresh parsley
- 2 cloves garlic, minced
- 1 teaspoon dried oregano
- 1/2 teaspoon salt
- 1/4 teaspoon black pepper
- 2 cups marinara sauce
- Fresh basil leaves for garnish

Instructions:

1. Preheat the oven to 400°F (200°C). Cut the spaghetti squash in half lengthwise and scoop out the seeds and membranes.

2. Place the squash halves cut-side down on a baking sheet and roast in the oven for about 40-50 minutes or until the flesh is tender.

3. While the squash is roasting, prepare the meatballs. In a large bowl, combine the ground beef or turkey, almond flour or breadcrumbs, grated Parmesan cheese, egg, chopped parsley, minced garlic, dried oregano, salt, and black pepper. Mix well until all ingredients are evenly incorporated.

4. Shape the mixture into small meatballs, about 1 inch in diameter.

5. Heat a skillet over medium heat and lightly grease it with olive oil. Cook the meatballs in batches until browned on all sides and cooked through, about 8-10 minutes. Remove from the skillet and set aside.

6. Once the spaghetti squash is cooked, use a fork to scrape the flesh into strands. Place the spaghetti squash strands in a large serving bowl.

7. Heat the marinara sauce in a saucepan over medium heat until warmed through.

8. Pour the marinara sauce over the spaghetti squash strands and toss to coat. Add the meatballs on top.

9. Garnish with fresh basil leaves and serve hot.

Baked Salmon with Dill Sauce

Ingredients:

- 4 salmon fillets
- 2 tablespoons olive oil
- 2 tablespoons fresh lemon juice
- 2 cloves garlic, minced
- 1 teaspoon dried dill
- 1/2 teaspoon salt
- 1/4 teaspoon black pepper

Dill Sauce:

- 1/2 cup Greek yogurt
- 1 tablespoon fresh dill, chopped
- 1 tablespoon fresh lemon juice
- 1 teaspoon Dijon mustard
- Salt and pepper to taste

Instructions:

1. Preheat the oven to 400°F (200°C). Line a baking sheet with parchment paper.

2. In a small bowl, whisk together the olive oil, lemon juice, minced garlic, dried dill, salt, and black pepper.

3. Place the salmon fillets on the prepared baking sheet. Brush the salmon with the lemon herb mixture, ensuring they are coated evenly.

4. Bake the salmon for about 12-15 minutes or until it flakes easily with a fork and reaches an internal temperature of 145°F (63°C).

5. While the salmon is baking, prepare the dill sauce. In a separate bowl, combine the Greek yogurt, chopped dill, lemon juice, Dijon mustard, salt, and pepper. Stir well to combine.

6. Once the salmon is cooked, remove it from the oven and let it rest for a few minutes. Serve the salmon hot with a dollop of dill sauce on top.

Turkey Chili with Sweet Potatoes

Ingredients:

- 1 tablespoon olive oil
- 1 onion, chopped
- 2 cloves garlic, minced
- 1 pound ground turkey
- 2 cups sweet potatoes, peeled and diced
- 1 red bell pepper, diced
- 1 can (15 ounces) diced tomatoes
- 1 can (15 ounces) kidney beans, rinsed and drained
- 1 cup low-sodium chicken or vegetable broth
- 2 tablespoons chili powder
- 1 teaspoon cumin
- 1/2 teaspoon paprika
- Salt and pepper to taste
- Optional toppings: chopped fresh cilantro, shredded cheese, plain Greek yogurt

Instructions:

1. Heat olive oil in a large pot or Dutch oven over medium heat. Add the chopped onion and minced

garlic, sauté for about 3-4 minutes until the onion is translucent and fragrant.

2. Add the ground turkey to the pot and cook until browned, breaking it up into smaller pieces with a spatula.

3. Stir in the diced sweet potatoes, red bell pepper, diced tomatoes, kidney beans, chicken or vegetable broth, chili powder, cumin, paprika, salt, and pepper.

4. Bring the chili to a boil, then reduce the heat and simmer uncovered for about 25-30 minutes, stirring occasionally, until the sweet potatoes are tender.

5. Taste and adjust the seasoning as needed. Serve the turkey chili hot, garnished with chopped fresh cilantro, shredded cheese, and a dollop of plain Greek yogurt if desired.

Roasted Cauliflower Steaks

Ingredients:

- 1 large head of cauliflower
- 2 tablespoons olive oil
- 2 cloves garlic, minced

- 1 teaspoon smoked paprika

- 1/2 teaspoon cumin

- 1/2 teaspoon turmeric

- Salt and pepper to taste

Instructions:

1. Preheat the oven to 425°F (220°C). Line a baking sheet with parchment paper.

2. Remove the leaves from the cauliflower head and trim the stem. Place the cauliflower head upright on a cutting board. Slice the cauliflower vertically into 1-inch thick steaks, starting from the center of the head.

3. In a small bowl, whisk together the olive oil, minced garlic, smoked paprika, cumin, turmeric, salt, and pepper.

4. Brush both sides of each cauliflower steak with the spice mixture, ensuring they are well coated.

5. Place the cauliflower steaks on the prepared baking sheet and roast in the oven for about 25-30 minutes, flipping them halfway through, until they are tender and golden brown.

6. Remove from the oven and let the cauliflower
    steaks cool for a few minutes before serving. Serve
    as a main dish with a side of quinoa or a salad.

Mexican Stuffed Zucchini Boats

Ingredients:

- 4 medium zucchinis
- 1 tablespoon olive oil
- 1 onion, chopped
- 2 cloves garlic, minced
- 1 red bell pepper, chopped
- 1 jalapeño pepper, seeds removed and minced (optional)
- 1 pound lean ground beef or turkey
- 1 cup cooked quinoa
- 1 can (15 ounces) black beans, rinsed and drained
- 1 cup diced tomatoes
- 1 teaspoon chili powder
- 1/2 teaspoon cumin
- Salt and pepper to taste
- Shredded cheddar cheese for topping (optional)
- Fresh cilantro leaves for garnish

Instructions:

1. Preheat the oven to 400°F (200°C). Cut the zucchinis in half lengthwise and scoop out the centers to create a hollow boat shape. Set the zucchini boats aside.

2. Heat olive oil in a large skillet over medium heat. Add the chopped onion, minced garlic, red bell pepper, and minced jalapeño pepper (if using). Sauté for about 5 minutes until the vegetables are tender.

3. Add the ground beef or turkey to the skillet and cook until browned, breaking it up into smaller pieces with a spatula.

4. Stir in the cooked quinoa, black beans, diced tomatoes, chili powder, cumin, salt, and pepper. Cook for an additional 2-3 minutes to allow the flavors to meld together.

5. Place the zucchini boats in a baking dish and spoon the meat and vegetable mixture into each boat, filling them generously.

6. Cover the baking dish with foil and bake in the preheated oven for about 25-30 minutes until the zucchini is tender.

7. Remove the foil and sprinkle the stuffed zucchini boats with shredded cheddar cheese, if desired. Return to the oven for an additional 5 minutes until the cheese is melted and bubbly.

8. Garnish with fresh cilantro leaves and serve hot.

Lemon Garlic Shrimp and Broccoli

Ingredients:

- 1 pound shrimp, peeled and deveined
- 1 tablespoon olive oil
- 4 cloves garlic, minced
- 1 teaspoon lemon zest
- 2 tablespoons fresh lemon juice
- 1/2 teaspoon dried oregano
- 1/4 teaspoon red pepper flakes (optional)
- Salt and pepper to taste
- 2 cups broccoli florets

Instructions:

1. Heat olive oil in a large skillet over medium heat. Add the minced garlic and sauté for about 1 minute until fragrant.

2. Add the shrimp to the skillet and cook for 2-3 minutes until they start to turn pink.

3. In a small bowl, whisk together the lemon zest, lemon juice, dried oregano, red pepper flakes (if using), salt, and pepper.

4. Pour the lemon mixture over the shrimp in the skillet and stir to coat the shrimp evenly. Cook for an additional 1-2 minutes until the shrimp are fully cooked and coated in the lemon garlic sauce.

5. Remove the shrimp from the skillet and set aside. Add the broccoli florets to the skillet and cook for about 4-5 minutes until they are tender-crisp.

6. Return the cooked shrimp to the skillet with the broccoli and toss everything together to combine.

7. Serve the lemon garlic shrimp and broccoli hot as a standalone dish or over a bed of cooked quinoa or cauliflower rice.

Quinoa-Stuffed Bell Peppers

Ingredients:

- 4 bell peppers (any color), tops removed and seeds removed
- 1 tablespoon olive oil
- 1 onion, chopped
- 2 cloves garlic, minced
- 1 zucchini, diced
- 1 cup cooked quinoa
- 1 can (15 ounces) diced tomatoes
- 1 can (15 ounces) black beans, rinsed and drained
- 1 teaspoon chili powder
- 1/2 teaspoon cumin
- Salt and pepper to taste
- Shredded Monterey Jack or cheddar cheese for topping (optional)
- Fresh cilantro leaves for garnish

Instructions:

1. Preheat the oven to 375°F (190°C). Place the bell peppers in a baking dish and set aside.

2. Heat olive oil in a large skillet over medium heat. Add the chopped onion, minced garlic, and diced zucchini. Sauté for about 5 minutes until the vegetables are tender.

3. Stir in the cooked quinoa, diced tomatoes, black beans, chili powder, cumin, salt, and pepper. Cook for an additional 2-3 minutes to allow the flavors to meld together.

4. Spoon the quinoa mixture into each bell pepper, filling them generously. If desired, sprinkle shredded Monterey Jack or cheddar cheese on top of each stuffed bell pepper.

5. Cover the baking dish with foil and bake in the preheated oven for about 30-35 minutes until the bell peppers are tender and the filling is heated through.

6. Remove the foil and bake for an additional 5 minutes until the cheese is melted and bubbly (if using).

7. Garnish with fresh cilantro leaves and serve the quinoa-stuffed bell peppers hot.

Baked Cod with Tomato and Olive Relish

Ingredients:

- 4 cod fillets
- 2 tablespoons olive oil
- 2 tablespoons fresh lemon juice
- 2 cloves garlic, minced
- 1 teaspoon dried oregano
- 1/2 teaspoon paprika
- Salt and pepper to taste

Tomato and Olive Relish:

- 1 cup cherry tomatoes, halved
- 1/4 cup Kalamata olives, pitted and chopped
- 2 tablespoons fresh basil leaves, chopped
- 1 tablespoon red wine vinegar
- 1 tablespoon olive oil
- Salt and pepper to taste

Instructions:

1. Preheat the oven to 400°F (200°C). Line a baking sheet with parchment paper.

2. Place the cod fillets on the prepared baking sheet. In a small bowl, whisk together the olive oil, lemon juice, minced garlic, dried oregano, paprika, salt, and pepper.

3. Brush the cod fillets with the lemon herb mixture, ensuring they are coated evenly.

4. Bake the cod in the preheated oven for about 12-15 minutes or until it flakes easily with a fork and reaches an internal temperature of 145°F (63°C).

5. While the cod is baking, prepare the tomato and olive relish. In a separate bowl, combine the halved cherry tomatoes, chopped Kalamata olives, chopped basil leaves, red wine vinegar, olive oil, salt, and pepper. Stir well to combine.

6. Once the cod is cooked, remove it from the oven and let it rest for a few minutes. Serve the baked cod hot with a spoonful of tomato and olive relish on top.

Chapter 5: Snacks and Appetizers

Enjoy these delicious and wholesome snacks and appetizers as part of your healthy PCOS diet.

Guacamole with Veggie Sticks

Ingredients:

- 2 ripe avocados
- 1 small onion, finely chopped
- 1 tomato, diced
- 1 jalapeño pepper, seeded and minced
- Juice of 1 lime
- 1 clove of garlic, minced
- Salt and pepper to taste
- Assorted veggie sticks (carrots, celery, bell peppers) for serving

Instructions:

1. Cut the avocados in half and remove the pits. Scoop out the flesh into a bowl.

2. Mash the avocado flesh with a fork until desired
    consistency.

3. Add the chopped onion, diced tomato, minced
    jalapeño pepper, lime juice, and minced garlic to the
    mashed avocado.

4. Season with salt and pepper to taste and mix well to
    combine all the ingredients.

5. Serve the guacamole with assorted veggie sticks for
    dipping.

Roasted Chickpeas

Ingredients:

- 1 can (15 oz) chickpeas, drained and rinsed
- 1 tablespoon olive oil
- 1 teaspoon ground cumin
- 1 teaspoon smoked paprika
- 1/2 teaspoon garlic powder
- 1/2 teaspoon sea salt
- 1/4 teaspoon cayenne pepper (optional)

Instructions:

1. Preheat the oven to 400°F (200°C) and line a baking sheet with parchment paper.

2. Pat dry the chickpeas with a clean kitchen towel to remove excess moisture.

3. In a bowl, toss the chickpeas with olive oil, ground cumin, smoked paprika, garlic powder, sea salt, and cayenne pepper (if using) until well coated.

4. Spread the seasoned chickpeas in a single layer on the prepared baking sheet.

5. Roast in the preheated oven for 25-30 minutes, or until the chickpeas are crispy and golden brown.

6. Remove from the oven and let cool slightly before serving as a crunchy snack.

Greek Yogurt Dip with Fresh Veggies

Ingredients:

- 1 cup Greek yogurt
- 1 tablespoon fresh lemon juice
- 1 clove garlic, minced
- 1 tablespoon chopped fresh dill
- Salt and pepper to taste

- Assorted fresh veggies (carrots, cucumbers, cherry tomatoes) for dipping

Instructions:

1. In a bowl, combine the Greek yogurt, fresh lemon juice, minced garlic, chopped dill, salt, and pepper.
2. Stir well until all the ingredients are thoroughly mixed.
3. Cover the bowl and refrigerate for at least 30 minutes to allow the flavors to meld.
4. Serve the Greek yogurt dip with assorted fresh veggies for a refreshing and healthy snack.

Cucumber and Hummus Roll-Ups

Ingredients:

- 1 large cucumber
- 1/2 cup hummus
- 1/4 cup finely diced red bell pepper
- 1/4 cup shredded carrot
- Fresh parsley leaves, for garnish

Instructions:

1. Slice the cucumber lengthwise into thin strips using a vegetable peeler or a mandoline slicer.
2. Spread a thin layer of hummus along the length of each cucumber strip.
3. Sprinkle diced red bell pepper and shredded carrot evenly over the hummus.
4. Roll up the cucumber strips tightly and secure with toothpicks if needed.
5. Garnish with fresh parsley leaves and serve as a light and refreshing appetizer.

Baked Sweet Potato Fries

Ingredients:

- 2 medium sweet potatoes, peeled and cut into thin fries
- 2 tablespoons olive oil
- 1 teaspoon paprika
- 1/2 teaspoon garlic powder
- 1/2 teaspoon sea salt
- Freshly ground black pepper to taste

Instructions:

1. Preheat the oven to 425°F (220°C) and line a baking sheet with parchment paper.

2. In a large bowl, toss the sweet potato fries with olive oil, paprika, garlic powder, sea salt, and black pepper until well coated.

3. Spread the seasoned sweet potato fries in a single layer on the prepared baking sheet.

4. Bake in the preheated oven for 20-25 minutes, or until the fries are crispy and golden brown, flipping halfway through.

5. Remove from the oven and let cool slightly before serving as a flavorful and nutritious snack.

Caprese Skewers

Ingredients:

- Cherry tomatoes

- Fresh mozzarella balls

- Fresh basil leaves

- Balsamic glaze

- Skewers or toothpicks

Instructions:

1. Thread one cherry tomato, one mozzarella ball, and
    one basil leaf onto each skewer or toothpick.
2. Repeat the process until all the ingredients are used.
3. Arrange the caprese skewers on a platter.
4. Drizzle with balsamic glaze for added flavor and
    presentation.
5. Serve as an elegant and bite-sized appetizer for any
    occasion.

Energy Bites with Nuts and Dates

Ingredients:

- 1 cup pitted dates
- 1 cup mixed nuts (almonds, walnuts, cashews)
- 2 tablespoons cocoa powder
- 1 tablespoon honey or maple syrup
- 1/2 teaspoon vanilla extract
- Shredded coconut (optional, for rolling)

Instructions:

1. Place the pitted dates, mixed nuts, cocoa powder,
    honey or maple syrup, and vanilla extract in a food
    processor.

2. Process until the ingredients are well combined and form a sticky mixture.

3. Scoop out tablespoon-sized portions of the mixture and roll into balls.

4. Optional: Roll the energy bites in shredded coconut for added texture and flavor.

5. Place the energy bites in an airtight container and refrigerate for at least 30 minutes to firm up.

6. Enjoy the energy bites as a healthy and energizing snack on the go.

Kale Chips

Ingredients:

- 1 bunch kale, washed and dried
- 1 tablespoon olive oil
- 1/2 teaspoon sea salt
- 1/4 teaspoon garlic powder
- 1/4 teaspoon smoked paprika (optional)

Instructions:

1. Preheat the oven to 300°F (150°C) and line a baking sheet with parchment paper.

2. Remove the tough stems from the kale leaves and tear the leaves into bite-sized pieces.

3. In a bowl, drizzle the kale leaves with olive oil and sprinkle with sea salt, garlic powder, and smoked paprika (if using).

4. Massage the kale leaves gently to evenly distribute the oil and seasonings.

5. Spread the seasoned kale leaves in a single layer on the prepared baking sheet.

6. Bake in the preheated oven for 15-20 minutes, or until the kale leaves are crispy and slightly browned.

7. Remove from the oven and let cool before enjoying the kale chips as a healthy and crunchy snack.

Spinach and Artichoke Dip

Ingredients:

- 1 cup frozen chopped spinach, thawed and drained
- 1 can (14 oz) artichoke hearts, drained and chopped
- 1 cup Greek yogurt
- 1/2 cup grated Parmesan cheese
- 1/2 cup shredded mozzarella cheese

- 1/4 cup mayonnaise

- 2 cloves garlic, minced

- 1/2 teaspoon onion powder

- Salt and pepper to taste

- Tortilla chips or pita bread for serving

Instructions:

1. Preheat the oven to 350°F (175°C).

2. In a bowl, combine the chopped spinach, chopped artichoke hearts, Greek yogurt, grated Parmesan cheese, shredded mozzarella cheese, mayonnaise, minced garlic, onion powder, salt, and pepper.

3. Mix well until all the ingredients are thoroughly combined.

4. Transfer the mixture to a baking dish and smooth the top.

5. Bake in the preheated oven for 20-25 minutes, or until the dip is hot and bubbly.

6. Remove from the oven and let cool slightly before serving with tortilla chips or pita bread.

Zucchini Fritters with Tzatziki Sauce

Ingredients:

- 2 medium zucchinis, grated
- 1 teaspoon salt
- 1/2 cup crumbled feta cheese
- 1/4 cup chopped fresh dill
- 2 green onions, finely chopped
- 2 eggs, lightly beaten
- 1/4 cup all-purpose flour
- 2 tablespoons olive oil
- Tzatziki sauce for serving

Instructions:

1. Place the grated zucchinis in a colander and sprinkle with salt. Let sit for 10 minutes to draw out excess moisture.
2. Squeeze the zucchinis to remove as much liquid as possible.
3. In a bowl, combine the grated zucchinis, crumbled feta cheese, chopped fresh dill, chopped green onions, beaten eggs, and all-purpose flour. Mix well to form a batter.

4. Heat olive oil in a skillet over medium heat.

5. Scoop spoonfuls of the zucchini batter into the hot skillet and flatten with the back of the spoon to form fritters.

6. Cook the fritters for 3-4 minutes per side, or until golden brown and crispy.

7. Remove from the skillet and place on a paper towel-lined plate to drain excess oil.

8. Serve the zucchini fritters warm with tzatziki sauce for dipping.

Flourless Chocolate Cake

Ingredients:

- 1 cup dark chocolate chips
- ½ cup unsalted butter
- ¾ cup granulated sugar
- 3 large eggs
- ½ cup unsweetened cocoa powder
- 1 teaspoon vanilla extract
- Pinch of salt
- Whipped cream, for serving (optional)
- Fresh berries, for garnish (optional)

Instructions:

1. Preheat your oven to 350°F (175°C) and grease a round cake pan.
2. In a microwave-safe bowl, melt the chocolate chips and butter together, stirring until smooth.
3. In a separate mixing bowl, whisk together the sugar, eggs, cocoa powder, vanilla extract, and salt.

4. Add the melted chocolate mixture to the bowl and stir until well combined.

5. Pour the batter into the prepared cake pan and smooth the top.

6. Bake in the preheated oven for 25-30 minutes or until a toothpick inserted into the center comes out with moist crumbs.

7. Remove the cake from the oven and let it cool in the pan for 10 minutes, then transfer it to a wire rack to cool completely.

8. Once cooled, serve the flourless chocolate cake with a dollop of whipped cream and fresh berries, if desired.

Berry Chia Pudding

Ingredients:

- 1 cup unsweetened almond milk
- ¼ cup chia seeds
- 1 tablespoon honey or maple syrup
- ½ teaspoon vanilla extract
- 1 cup mixed berries (strawberries, blueberries, raspberries)

Instructions:

1. In a jar or bowl, combine the almond milk, chia seeds, honey or maple syrup, and vanilla extract. Stir well.

2. Let the mixture sit for 5 minutes, then stir again to break up any clumps of chia seeds.

3. Cover the jar or bowl and refrigerate for at least 2 hours or overnight to allow the chia seeds to thicken.

4. Before serving, give the chia pudding a good stir to make sure it's evenly thickened.

5. Divide the pudding into serving bowls or glasses and top with mixed berries.

6. Enjoy the berry chia pudding as a healthy and refreshing dessert or breakfast.

Almond Butter Cookies

Ingredients:

- 1 cup almond butter
- ⅔ cup granulated sugar
- 1 large egg
- 1 teaspoon vanilla extract

- ½ teaspoon baking soda

- Pinch of salt

- ½ cup dark chocolate chips (optional)

Instructions:

1. Preheat your oven to 350°F (175°C) and line a baking sheet with parchment paper.

2. In a mixing bowl, combine the almond butter, sugar, egg, vanilla extract, baking soda, and salt. Stir until well combined.

3. If desired, fold in the dark chocolate chips to add extra flavor and texture to the cookies.

4. Scoop tablespoon-sized portions of dough and roll them into balls. Place the balls onto the prepared baking sheet, spacing them about 2 inches apart.

5. Gently press down on each dough ball with a fork to create a crisscross pattern.

6. Bake in the preheated oven for 10-12 minutes or until the edges are golden brown.

7. Remove the cookies from the oven and let them cool on the baking sheet for 5 minutes, then transfer them to a wire rack to cool completely.

8. Enjoy the almond butter cookies as a delicious and wholesome treat.

Greek Yogurt Berry Parfait

Ingredients:

- 1 cup Greek yogurt
- 2 tablespoons honey or maple syrup
- 1 teaspoon vanilla extract
- 1 cup mixed berries (strawberries, blueberries, raspberries)
- ¼ cup granola

Instructions:

1. In a small bowl, mix together the Greek yogurt, honey or maple syrup, and vanilla extract.
2. Layer the yogurt mixture, mixed berries, and granola in a glass or parfait dish, starting with a dollop of yogurt at the bottom.
3. Repeat the layers until all the ingredients are used, finishing with a sprinkle of granola on top.
4. Serve the Greek yogurt berry parfait immediately or refrigerate for later.

5. Enjoy the creamy and fruity parfait as a satisfying dessert or breakfast option.

Pumpkin Spice Muffins

Ingredients:

- 1 ½ cups all-purpose flour
- 1 teaspoon baking powder
- ½ teaspoon baking soda
- 1 teaspoon ground cinnamon
- ½ teaspoon ground ginger
- ¼ teaspoon ground nutmeg
- ¼ teaspoon ground cloves
- ¼ teaspoon salt
- ½ cup granulated sugar
- ½ cup packed brown sugar
- ½ cup pumpkin puree
- ¼ cup unsweetened applesauce
- 2 large eggs
- 1 teaspoon vanilla extract

Instructions:

1. Preheat your oven to 350°F (175°C) and line a muffin tin with paper liners.
2. In a mixing bowl, whisk together the flour, baking powder, baking soda, cinnamon, ginger, nutmeg, cloves, and salt.
3. In a separate bowl, mix together the granulated sugar, brown sugar, pumpkin puree, applesauce, eggs, and vanilla extract until well combined.
4. Gradually add the dry ingredients to the wet ingredients, stirring until just combined. Do not overmix.
5. Divide the batter evenly among the muffin cups, filling each about ¾ full.
6. Bake in the preheated oven for 18-20 minutes or until a toothpick inserted into the center of a muffin comes out clean.
7. Remove the muffins from the oven and let them cool in the tin for 5 minutes, then transfer them to a wire rack to cool completely.
8. Enjoy the pumpkin spice muffins as a delightful fall treat.

Coconut Macaroons

Ingredients:

- 2 cups shredded coconut (unsweetened)
- ½ cup sweetened condensed milk
- 1 teaspoon vanilla extract
- Pinch of salt
- 2 large egg whites
- Optional: Dark chocolate, melted (for drizzling)

Instructions:

1. Preheat your oven to 325°F (160°C) and line a baking sheet with parchment paper.
2. In a mixing bowl, combine the shredded coconut, sweetened condensed milk, vanilla extract, and salt. Stir until well mixed.
3. In a separate bowl, whisk the egg whites until they form stiff peaks.
4. Gently fold the beaten egg whites into the coconut mixture until evenly combined.
5. Using a tablespoon or a small cookie scoop, drop mounds of the mixture onto the prepared baking sheet, spacing them about 1 inch apart.

6. Bake in the preheated oven for 20-25 minutes or until the macaroons are golden brown on the edges.

7. Remove the macaroons from the oven and let them cool on the baking sheet for 5 minutes, then transfer them to a wire rack to cool completely.

8. For an extra touch, drizzle melted dark chocolate over the cooled macaroons.

9. Enjoy the chewy and coconutty macaroons as a delightful sweet treat.

Baked Apples with Cinnamon

Ingredients:

- 4 apples (Granny Smith or Honeycrisp)
- 2 tablespoons unsalted butter, melted
- 2 tablespoons honey or maple syrup
- 1 teaspoon ground cinnamon
- ¼ teaspoon ground nutmeg
- ¼ teaspoon ground cloves
- Optional toppings: Chopped nuts, raisins, or a dollop of Greek yogurt

Instructions:

1. Preheat your oven to 375°F (190°C) and grease a baking dish.
2. Core the apples, leaving the bottoms intact, and peel a strip of skin around the top of each apple.
3. Place the cored apples in the greased baking dish.
4. In a small bowl, mix together the melted butter, honey or maple syrup, cinnamon, nutmeg, and cloves.
5. Drizzle the butter mixture over the apples, making sure to coat them evenly.
6. Bake in the preheated oven for 30-35 minutes or until the apples are tender and slightly caramelized.
7. Remove the baked apples from the oven and let them cool for a few minutes.
8. Serve the baked apples as is or sprinkle them with chopped nuts, raisins, or a dollop of Greek yogurt for added flavor and texture.
9. Enjoy the warm and comforting baked apples as a wholesome dessert or snack.

Chocolate Avocado Mousse

Ingredients:

- 2 ripe avocados
- ½ cup unsweetened cocoa powder
- ½ cup maple syrup or honey
- ¼ cup unsweetened almond milk or coconut milk
- 1 teaspoon vanilla extract
- Pinch of salt
- Optional toppings: Shredded coconut, sliced almonds, or fresh berries

Instructions:

1. Scoop the flesh of the ripe avocados into a blender or food processor.
2. Add the cocoa powder, maple syrup or honey, almond milk or coconut milk, vanilla extract, and salt to the blender.
3. Blend all the ingredients together until smooth and creamy, scraping down the sides as needed.
4. Taste the chocolate avocado mousse and adjust the sweetness or cocoa intensity if desired.

5. Transfer the mousse to serving dishes or glasses and refrigerate for at least 1 hour to allow it to chill and set.

6. Before serving, garnish the mousse with shredded coconut, sliced almonds, or fresh berries.

7. Enjoy the rich and indulgent chocolate avocado mousse as a healthier alternative to traditional chocolate desserts.

Lemon Poppy Seed Loaf

Ingredients:

- 2 cups all-purpose flour
- 1 ½ teaspoons baking powder
- ½ teaspoon baking soda
- ¼ teaspoon salt
- ½ cup unsalted butter, softened
- 1 cup granulated sugar
- 2 large eggs
- 1 teaspoon vanilla extract
- 1 tablespoon lemon zest
- 2 tablespoons fresh lemon juice
- ¾ cup Greek yogurt

- 2 tablespoons poppy seeds

Instructions:

1. Preheat your oven to 350°F (175°C) and grease a loaf pan.
2. In a mixing bowl, whisk together the flour, baking powder, baking soda, and salt.
3. In a separate large bowl, cream together the softened butter and granulated sugar until light and fluffy.
4. Beat in the eggs, one at a time, followed by the vanilla extract, lemon zest, and lemon juice.
5. Gradually add the dry ingredients to the wet ingredients, alternating with the Greek yogurt, beginning and ending with the dry ingredients. Mix until just combined.
6. Fold in the poppy seeds, making sure they are evenly distributed throughout the batter.
7. Pour the batter into the greased loaf pan and smooth the top with a spatula.

8. Bake in the preheated oven for 50-60 minutes or until a toothpick inserted into the center of the loaf comes out clean.

9. Remove the lemon poppy seed loaf from the oven and let it cool in the pan for 10 minutes, then transfer it to a wire rack to cool completely.

10. Slice the loaf and serve it as a delightful citrus-infused dessert or breakfast bread.

Vanilla Berry Nice Cream

Ingredients:

- 4 ripe bananas, peeled and frozen
- 1 cup mixed berries (strawberries, blueberries, raspberries)
- 1 teaspoon vanilla extract
- Optional toppings: Fresh berries, crushed nuts, or shredded coconut

Instructions:

1. Place the frozen bananas, mixed berries, and vanilla extract in a blender or food processor.

2. Blend the ingredients on high speed until smooth and creamy, scraping down the sides as needed.

3. If the mixture is too thick, add a splash of almond milk or coconut milk to help with blending.

4. Once the nice cream reaches a soft-serve consistency, transfer it to a freezer-safe container.

5. Freeze the nice cream for at least 1 hour or until it firms up.

6. Before serving, let the nice cream sit at room temperature for a few minutes to soften slightly.

7. Scoop the vanilla berry nice cream into bowls or cones and garnish with fresh berries, crushed nuts, or shredded coconut if desired.

8. Enjoy the refreshing and guilt-free vanilla berry nice cream as a healthier alternative to traditional ice cream.

Chapter 7: Beverages

Enjoy these refreshing and flavorful beverages as part of your PCOS diet journey. They will not only quench your thirst but also provide nourishment and support for your overall well-being

Green Detox Smoothie

Ingredients:

- 1 cup spinach leaves
- 1 green apple, cored and chopped
- 1 ripe banana
- ½ cucumber, peeled and chopped
- 1 tablespoon fresh lemon juice
- 1 tablespoon chia seeds
- 1 cup unsweetened almond milk
- Ice cubes (optional)

Instructions:

1. In a blender, combine the spinach, green apple, banana, cucumber, lemon juice, chia seeds, and almond milk.

2. Blend on high speed until smooth and creamy.

3. If desired, add a few ice cubes and blend again until chilled.

4. Pour the green detox smoothie into a glass and serve immediately. Enjoy the refreshing and nourishing flavors!

Turmeric Golden Milk

Ingredients:

- 2 cups unsweetened almond milk
- 1 teaspoon ground turmeric
- ½ teaspoon ground cinnamon
- ¼ teaspoon ground ginger
- 1 tablespoon honey or maple syrup
- 1 teaspoon coconut oil
- Pinch of black pepper

Instructions:

1. In a small saucepan, heat the almond milk over
    medium heat until hot but not boiling.
2. Add the turmeric, cinnamon, ginger, honey or
    maple syrup, coconut oil, and black pepper to the
    saucepan.
3. Whisk the mixture until well combined and heated
    through.
4. Remove from heat and pour the turmeric golden
    milk into mugs.
5. Stir well before serving. Savor the warm and
    comforting flavors of this nourishing beverage.

Berry Blast Smoothie

Ingredients:

- 1 cup mixed berries (strawberries, blueberries,
  raspberries)
- 1 ripe banana
- ½ cup plain Greek yogurt
- 1 tablespoon honey or agave syrup
- 1 cup unsweetened almond milk
- Ice cubes (optional)

Instructions:

1. Place the mixed berries, ripe banana, Greek yogurt, honey or agave syrup, and almond milk in a blender.
2. Blend until smooth and creamy.
3. If desired, add a few ice cubes and blend again until chilled.
4. Pour the berry blast smoothie into glasses and serve immediately. Enjoy the burst of fruity goodness!

Iced Herbal Tea with Citrus

Ingredients:

- 4 cups water
- 4 herbal tea bags (such as chamomile, peppermint, or hibiscus)
- 1 lemon, sliced
- 1 lime, sliced
- Fresh mint leaves (optional)
- Ice cubes

Instructions:

1. Bring the water to a boil in a saucepan.

2. Add the herbal tea bags and let steep for 5-10 minutes.

3. Remove the tea bags and allow the tea to cool to room temperature.

4. Once cooled, transfer the tea to a pitcher and add the lemon and lime slices.

5. For extra flavor, you can also add fresh mint leaves.

6. Refrigerate the pitcher for at least 2 hours to allow the flavors to infuse.

7. Serve the iced herbal tea over ice cubes. Sip and feel refreshed with every citrusy sip!

Cucumber and Mint Infused Water

Ingredients:

- 1 cucumber, thinly sliced
- Handful of fresh mint leaves
- 8 cups water
- Ice cubes

Instructions:

1. In a large pitcher, combine the cucumber slices and fresh mint leaves.

2. Pour the water over the cucumber and mint.

3. Place the pitcher in the refrigerator and let it infuse for at least 1 hour.

4. When ready to serve, add ice cubes to individual glasses and pour the cucumber and mint infused water over the ice.

5. Enjoy the crisp and refreshing taste of this revitalizing beverage!

Energizing Matcha Latte

Ingredients:

- 1 teaspoon matcha powder
- 1 tablespoon hot water
- 1 cup unsweetened almond milk
- 1 teaspoon honey or maple syrup

Instructions:

1. In a small bowl, whisk the matcha powder and hot water together until smooth and frothy.

2. In a saucepan, heat the almond milk over medium heat until hot but not boiling.

3. Pour the hot almond milk into a mug and add the matcha mixture.

4. Stir in the honey or maple syrup until well combined.

5. Sip and savor the invigorating flavors of this energizing matcha latte.

Refreshing Watermelon Cooler

Ingredients:

- 4 cups cubed watermelon
- Juice of 1 lime
- 1 tablespoon fresh mint leaves, chopped
- Ice cubes

Instructions:

1. Place the cubed watermelon, lime juice, and fresh mint leaves in a blender.

2. Blend until smooth and well combined.

3. If desired, add a few ice cubes and blend again until chilled.

4. Pour the refreshing watermelon cooler into glasses and garnish with mint leaves.

5. Take a sip and experience the cool and hydrating sensation of this summery beverage.

Blueberry Lemonade

Ingredients:

- 1 cup fresh or frozen blueberries
- Juice of 4 lemons
- 4 cups water
- ¼ cup honey or agave syrup
- Ice cubes

Instructions:

1. In a blender, combine the blueberries, lemon juice, water, and honey or agave syrup.
2. Blend until smooth and well mixed.
3. Strain the mixture through a fine-mesh sieve into a pitcher to remove any pulp or seeds.
4. Chill the blueberry lemonade in the refrigerator for at least 1 hour.
5. Serve over ice cubes and enjoy the tangy and sweet combination of blueberries and lemons.

Spiced Apple Cider

Ingredients:

- 4 cups apple cider
- 2 cinnamon sticks
- 4 whole cloves
- 1 orange, sliced
- 1 tablespoon honey or maple syrup (optional)

Instructions:

1. In a saucepan, combine the apple cider, cinnamon sticks, whole cloves, and orange slices.
2. Bring the mixture to a simmer over medium heat.
3. Reduce the heat to low and let the spiced apple cider simmer for 10-15 minutes.
4. If desired, stir in honey or maple syrup for added sweetness.
5. Remove from heat and strain the spiced apple cider into mugs.
6. Sip and enjoy the cozy and fragrant flavors of this comforting beverage.

Coconut Water Electrolyte Drink

Ingredients:

- 2 cups coconut water
- Juice of 1 lemon
- Juice of 1 lime
- 2 tablespoons honey or agave syrup
- Pinch of sea salt

Instructions:

1. In a pitcher, combine the coconut water, lemon juice, lime juice, honey or agave syrup, and sea salt.
2. Stir well until the ingredients are thoroughly mixed.
3. Chill the coconut water electrolyte drink in the refrigerator for at least 30 minutes.
4. Serve in glasses with ice cubes for a revitalizing and hydrating beverage.

CONCLUSION

As we come to the end of this journey through the "Easy PCOS Diet Cookbook," it's time to reflect on the valuable knowledge and delicious recipes we've explored together. In Chapter 9, aptly titled "Conclusion," we will recap the key takeaways, discuss the importance of maintaining a healthy PCOS diet beyond the cookbook, express final thoughts and encouragement, provide additional resources for PCOS support, and acknowledge those who have contributed to the creation of this cookbook.

Recap of Key Takeaways

Throughout the preceding chapters, we delved into various aspects of the PCOS diet and how it can positively impact those with Polycystic Ovary Syndrome. We learned about the importance of choosing nutrient-dense foods, incorporating whole grains, lean proteins, and healthy fats, while limiting processed foods and refined sugars. We discovered the benefits of balancing macronutrients and managing portion sizes to promote stable blood sugar levels. Moreover, we explored the significance of consuming high-fiber foods, antioxidant-rich fruits and vegetables, and incorporating regular exercise into our lifestyle.

Maintaining a Healthy PCOS Diet beyond the Cookbook

While this cookbook has provided you with a wide array of delectable recipes, it's crucial to recognize that a healthy PCOS diet extends beyond the pages of this book. Embracing a sustainable lifestyle change is key to long-term success in managing PCOS symptoms. By making mindful choices at the grocery store, incorporating physical activity into your daily routine, and seeking support from healthcare professionals or support groups, you can continue to nourish your body and manage your PCOS effectively.

Final Thoughts and Encouragement

Embarking on a new dietary journey, particularly one tailored to manage a health condition like PCOS, can feel overwhelming at times. It's essential to approach this process with patience, self-compassion, and a sense of adventure. Remember that every small step you take towards a healthier lifestyle is a step in the right direction. Celebrate your successes, learn from any setbacks, and continue to prioritize your well-being.

www.ingramcontent.com/pod-product-compliance
Lightning Source LLC
Chambersburg PA
CBHW050032260726

48658CB00005B/1571